Quick & Easy Physical Fitness For Everyone
(No Matter The Challenge)

By
Stanley W. Morey, Ph.D.

Acknowledgements

This book would not have been possible without the editorial skills and help with the photos by my wife Gery Morey. I also want to thank Liz Lamagese for making my files available to Amazon. I thank them very much for their assistance. I also wish to thank Robby Robinson (Masters Mr. Olympia), who woke me from the doldrums of my Multiple Myeloma diagnosis, and made me design a fitness program for myself at home.

Prologue

The main reason for this book is because my Multiple Myeloma has not allowed me to visit a gym or health club in a number of years. In order to have some semblance of fitness, I had to devise exercises that I could do at home. Earlier in my life I owned a Health Club, and was a competitive bodybuilder, so staying in shape was in my blood. Training was an essential part of my life and I was determined not to let a health issue interfere with my physical fitness. In my case, a health challenge prevented me from training at a gym. For the average person, exercising at a health club is challenging due to busy schedules and time constraints. I designed this book for the average person to work out at home, and possibly work up to visiting a health club. These exercises have worked for me, and I am sure they will work for you.

Stanley W. Morey, Ph.D.

Chapter 1. Physical Fitness

A. What is Physical Fitness?

Is jogging a fad? Will it pass into history like the hula-hoop? What about being physically fit? Is it a fad also? In 1960, no one had any idea about the number of people jogging regularly. In 1972, the number of regular joggers was estimated to be about 6 million. This number jumped to 11 million in 1975 and to 17 million in 1978. Today it is estimated that about 10 million people play tennis regularly and another 3.1 million play racquetball. There is no doubt that the commercial health clubs are cashing in on this fitness explosion.

Why do people exercise daily? Are they lacking some element of common sense? (If they are, there are over 35 million individuals in the United States afflicted with the same abnormality.) Some people exercise because the commercial sector of our society has made it mandatory for "attractive" people to be thin; others exercise because they are concerned with achieving some ideal body shape; still others do it because they are interested in developing certain muscles or bodybuilding. Whatever the initial reason, most of these individuals soon realize the benefits of regular, daily exercise. They are well aware that the lack of exercise is directly or indirectly related to the development of coronary heart disease, hypertension, obesity, anxiety, depression, and lower back pain and they are now exercising to improve their general physical and mental health. Consequently, many people desire some degree of physical fitness.

 However, obesity and diabetes as well as other abnormalities due to being overweight are rampant in our society. Obesity in the young has become epidemic, and as a society we appear to accept the fact that people are overweight. Physical fitness for the general population seems to be non-existent; it appears that all the advertisements for fitness equipment, and losing weight are doing absolutely nothing. Why is this occurring? Maybe, our sedentary lifestyles, computer games lack of physical education in our schools are the culprit? Only a small minority appears to heed the advice of fitness experts, and is physically fit. Our busy lifestyles may leave us little time to exercise or join a health club, and our consumption of refined, and junk foods needs to stop. We need to start putting physical fitness higher on our agendas, making it a priority in our lives.

But what is physical fitness? Physical fitness is very individualistic. Each person has a different set of needs and desires. For example a professional athlete requires a different degree of fitness than a businessperson. And choosing the level of fitness that fits your life style will come as you progress with your exercise program.   As you progress with your exercising, you will begin to feel both physically and mentally better. Plus you will develop a better self-image. And you will be closer to or at your ideal body weight. Your cardiovascular endurance will improve and your muscular strength, endurance, and flexibility will also improve. (Self-evaluation techniques and norms will be given throughout this chapter to help you determine your fitness.) Physical fitness is composed of a number of components, some of which are more important than others are. The degree of importance is determined by your occupational and recreational pursuits.

HEALTH-RELATED COMPONENTS	PERFORMANCE-RELATED COMPONENTS
Muscular strength	Agility
Muscular endurance	Speed
Flexibility	Neuromuscular condition
Body composition	Specific skills
Cardiovascular endurance	

This list is not exhaustive. Many other components can be included but their value is questionable.

The value of each health related component and the specific way to develop each of them will be explained, but first you should understand something about what happens to the body when you put it under the stress of physical activity.

B. What Happens to the Body During Exercise?

When you exercise a number of different systems begin to work harder to supply the energy needed to perform the physical activity. The muscular, neuromuscular, circulatory, and respiratory systems all respond to this new energy demand. Every movement you make is made possible by the contraction of over 600 muscles, some of which are connected, to over 250 bones. These muscles perform many different functions, such as propelling food along the digestive tract (peristalsis), taking air into the lungs, constricting blood vessels, and propelling blood throughout the body.

There are three types of muscles: striated, smooth, and cardiac. Striated muscles are attached to bone and compose most of the body's musculature. They are responsible for movement of the skeletal system, and can only constrict if they are stimulated from an external source, such as the brain. Smooth muscles are those of the gut and other internal organs of the body and do not require external stimulation. They are responsible for movement within the body, such as peristalsis. The cardiac muscle makes up the heart and is responsible for pumping blood through the blood vessels. It does not require external stimulation because the heart can send out its own impulse that will cause its own muscle fibers to contract.

In order for all three types of muscle to contract, they need some form of energy. Just as an automobile needs gasoline and oxygen before it can run, the body needs fuel, called adenosine-tri-phosphate (ATP), and oxygen before it can run. The body gets the oxygen through the lungs. In the lungs oxygen comes in close contact with blood that moves through very tiny thin arteries called alveoli. Here the blood picks up the needed oxygen and transports it to all the cells of the body. When the oxygen enters the cell, some waste products (carbon dioxide and water) from the production of energy in the cell (energy metabolism) are taken up by the blood and then transported back through the veins where it is exhaled by the lungs, and as water through the kidneys. Along with oxygen, ATP is required to produce the energy necessary for all bodily functions. ATP is the energy currency of the body. When the body breaks it down, it liberates energy.

Energy production, which occurs in the presence of an adequate supply of oxygen, is called aerobic metabolism. As aerobic metabolism continues, the body reaches a point where it can no longer supply the needed oxygen necessary to breakdown foodstuffs and then it must resort to another form of energy production called anaerobic metabolism. Anaerobic metabolism utilizes the body's stored energy sources that can be broken down in the absence of oxygen. This is very costly, requiring lots of energy and the body can only perform at this level for short periods of time.

The way to increase the capacity of the aerobic system is by engaging in endurance type activities. Many exercises, such as, jogging, walking, swimming, bicycling, aerobic dancing, jumping rope, etc., can be endurance in nature. The key is to perform them in the correct manner, for a sufficient amount of time, and at an adequate intensity.

Some activities require anaerobic metabolism. Short, very intense exercise, such as running 100 meters as fast as you can, requires a large amount of energy in a short period of time. This energy cannot be supplied through the use of oxygen. Consequently the anaerobic system must supply the energy. Athletes and those people wishing to compete at high levels of competition benefit most from anaerobic training. Anaerobic training is hard and painful and not very practical for individuals who only wish to improve their fitness. Weightlifting also requires anaerobic energy; however, weight lifting and resistance exercises are very important in a total fitness program. Since weightlifting is primarily an anaerobic activity, you may wonder how weightlifters manage to work out for over an hour. Well, during an anaerobic workout something called oxygen debt is accumulated. Once an activity that is performed anaerobically is over, the body consumes extra oxygen to pay off or rebuild all the ATP utilized during the activity. When you lift weights, lift for less than a minute and then rest for a brief period. During this rest the oxygen debt is being repaid. If the rest period does not occur, you will only be able to lift weights for a short period of time.

C. Results of Inactivity

Modern living has made strenuous exercise less practical. Research has shown that even though modern human beings consume less food than their ancestors did, obesity is much more prevalent today than it was in the past. Why is this? It seems that though our ancestors were not on a regular exercise program and didn't lift weights at the local gym, their lives were filled with strenuous activities that consumed many calories and kept their heart, lungs, and circulatory and muscular systems in good condition. Today, with the advent of automation, our lifestyles are more sedentary and with this inactivity come obesity and a lack of fitness. (Our muscles were meant to be used and when they're not or not used enough, they begin to deteriorate.) Many individuals try to correct this situation through dieting only and drastically cut down their calorie intake, usually sacrificing vitamins and minerals needed for proper health. Others may throw themselves into a rigorous workout, after years of inactivity, instead of gradually incorporating exercise into their daily routines, possibly placing themselves at risk for a heart attack, stroke, or injury. The most sensible approach is to improve your nutritional status, by eating the proper foods, combined with a regular exercise regime.

D. Results of Regular, Adequate Exercise

Through a properly designed and executed exercise program, which includes cardiovascular endurance, muscular strength, endurance, and flexibility training, certain beneficial changes occur that are both physiological and psychological. The exact change that occurs will depend on the type of training/exercise you are performing. This is known as the principle of specificity of training. For example, if a person is only lifting heavy weights, he/she will obtain the benefit of greater muscular strength and size but will not gain much cardiovascular endurance or flexibility. Conversely, a jogger who performs little else gains the cardiovascular benefits but not muscle strength. Therefore, a well rounded, fitness program will encompass both strength/physique enhancement and cardiovascular endurance.

1. CARDIOVASCULAR ENDURANCE BENEFITS

    A. Decrease in resting heart rate.

    B. Decrease in exercise heart rate of submaximal workloads.

    C. Increase in the amount of blood the heart can pump

each beat (stroke volume).

D. Increase in lung capacity and, therefore, a decrease in the amount of breaths required during exercise and other strenuous activities.

E. Decreased blood pressure.

F. Increase in the ease of oxygen transportation from lungs to blood and from blood to tissue.

G. Increase in the maximal amount of oxygen the body can take in and utilize during maximal effort. (This is the best indicator of cardiovascular fitness)

H. Decrease in recovery time for the cardiovascular system and the body as a whole after strenuous effort.

I. Increase in cardiovascular efficiency.

J. Increase in protection from illness and disease.

K. Improved self-image.

L. Decrease in tension and increased ability to relax.

2. MUSCLE STRENGTH AND ENDURANCE BENEFITS

A. Increase in strength and endurance.

B. Increase in coordination.

C. Increase in size of the muscle mass (especially the strength training programs).

D. Increased protection from injuries.

E. Improved posture.

F. Decrease in chronic fatigue.

G. Improved physical appearance.

H. Improved self-image.

I. Increased muscular efficiency.

A strength program will increase muscular endurance as well as strength. However, a program designed just for muscular endurance will have much greater benefits.

3. FLEXIBILITY BENEFITS

A. Increased joint mobility and flexibility.

B. Decrease in minor aches, pains, stiffness, and soreness.

C. Improved ability to relax and reduce tension.

D. Greater protection from injuries.

E. Improved posture.

4. OVERALL REDUCTION OF RISK FACTORS

A total fitness program can help to reduce or eliminate a wide variety of health risk factors. For example, cardiovascular exercise can help to eliminate hypertension, hyperlipidemia, and smoking. Perhaps exercise makes the individual become more aware of his/her body and what is being put into it. Exercise can also lead to a reduction in body weight and stress, and can be a prime ingredient in the prevention of coronary heart disease.

Chapter 2. Exercise Program

A. Before Starting An Exercise Program

Before increasing your physical activity, you need to sit down and self-evaluate your present physical condition. Do you have any chronic pain, especially in the lower back? Do you have pains in the chest area? Are you extremely overweight? Do you smoke cigarettes? Do you have a persistent cough? Do you have unexplained bleeding or other discharges? If you answered "yes" to any of these questions, or have any questions about your health you should see a physician before increasing your activity level. It is advisable for anyone over the age of 40 to have a regular check-up and if you are over 35 years of age and have been inactive for the past few years you should also consult with a physician before starting any exercise program. And remember there is no age limit for starting an exercise program!

Everyone who is increasing his or her level of activity should do so gradually. This is especially true if you are physically inactive or overweight. I recommend that if you are among this group of individuals you begin with a brisk walking program for a month or more so that you can improve your cardiovascular endurance. Once you've become acclimated to the brisk walking, you may then begin some muscular strength and endurance improvement exercises. The first thing to do is to pick a time of day that best suits your likes and schedule. Many people find it more convenient to exercise in the late afternoon or evening. However, research has shown that since exercise acts as a stimulant, you should allow yourself two to four hours between the conclusion of exercise and attempting to sleep. (I personally exercise early in the morning.) But whatever time you choose, don't rush. Give yourself 45 minutes to an hour to exercise. Here are some general rules to help you make your exercise sessions more enjoyable.

Do not exercise immediately after a heavy meal.

The best time to exercise is about one hour before your next meal or two hours after the last one. You may find that you need up to four hours after a meal before exercising.

Start out your exercise program with light, easy exercises and progress steadily and slowly.

Start each exercise session with stretching exercises and easy warm-up activities. Start slowly and pick up the tempo 5 to 10 minutes into the session. Don't stop strenuous exercises suddenly. Cool down by exercising at a light intensity for the last 10 minutes of your program. Use light stretching exercises to finish your daily program. Never exercise if you have a fever or feel bloated or when your stomach is upset. Never try to "run through" or exercise through pain.

Listen to your body – it is trying to tell you something.

B. Cardiovascular Endurance

The number one killer in the world today is coronary heart disease (CHD). In the United States, it accounts for over half of all reported deaths and it is estimated that over 600,000 Americans between the ages of 25 and 65 died of CHD last year. That's more than the next three most common causes of death combined.

What can be done to help reduce or eliminate this disease from our society? Researchers have been working on this for decades and they have come up with a set of "risk factors" that are correlated to the incidence of CHD. Researchers are not stating that any one of these factors is the cause of CHD but if any of these combinations of factors are present the likelihood of developing CHD are doubled or even tripled.

1. **High blood pressure**. Elevated blood pressure can cause damage to the cardiovascular system and other vital organs. This damage leads to clots and thrombi, which can cause strokes and heart attacks. It is estimated that as many millions of Americans suffer unknowingly from hypertension.

2. **Hyperlipidemia (High Fat Levels).** The exact role of high cholesterol levels in the blood stream in the genesis of heart disease is controversial. It is currently believed that not all forms of cholesterol are harmful; in fact, the liver produces a large amount of cholesterol that the body uses in the manufacturing of sex hormones and other vital substances.

Researchers now feel that another form of cholesterol called Very Low Density Lipoproteins (LDL's), which cause the building of material (plaque) on the arterial walls. This build up of plaque reduces the amount of blood that can pass through; if the reduced blood flow is to a part of the heart, the result can be a heart attack or myocardial infarction. Another form of cholesterol, High Density Lipoproteins (HDL's) is believed to be a protector against this plaque buildup.

3. **Smoking.** It is hard to believe that so many people still smoke after it has been proven that smoking causes cancer and coronary heart disease not to mention the complications experienced by the fetuses of smoking females. When a person smokes, the harmful substances contained in the smoke enter the blood steam via the lungs. These substances then irritate the lining of the arteries, which leads to the buildup of plaque, which in turn leads to reduced blood flow to the heart muscle.

Other risk factors are:

4. Obesity   5. Stress 6. Inactivity   7. Diabetes

Some risk factors cannot be reduced but are still of concern when determining a person's likelihood of developing CHD.

1. Age   2. Sex 3. Race 4. Genetic factors/family history

What can you do to reduce or eliminate some of these risk Factors? The adjunct of a regular exercise program, will definitely help you reduce or control many of these risk factors. A regular exercise program will not only eliminate the risk factor of inactivity, it will also help to eliminate the risk factor caused by obesity. Exercise also increases the level of HDL's, which help combat the formation of plaque in the blood stream, plus reduces blood pressure in people with hypertension. The hardest part of an exercise program is picking out the cardiovascular endurance exercise. There are many exercises, activities, and sports that can be cardiovascular. These are defined as aerobics. More information can be obtained from a book entitled Aerobics, by Dr. Kenneth Cooper. The following list covers some of the better-known cardiovascular endurance activities.

1. Jogging
2. Swimming
3. Bicycling
4. Rope jumping
5. Aerobic dancing
6. Basketball
7. Racquetball
8. Handball
9. Tennis
10. Volleyball

C. Intensity of Exercise

How hard should you perform an exercise for it to add to your cardiovascular endurance? Research has shown that an intensity of 50 to 80 percent of your maximal effort is considered optimal. How do you determine the amount of effort? Your heart rate is the best approach. During exercise your heart rate should get up to 65 to 85 percent of its maximal beats per minute. To determine this, first determine your maximal heart rate. Taking 220 minus your age can make a good guess. Next, determine your resting heart rate. The best way to do this is to count your pulse rate for 30 seconds and then multiply that number by two. This should be done upon awaking in the morning and while still in bed. Finally, subtract your resting heart rate from your maximal heart rate. This will give you your heart rate reserve. Example: A 50-year-old individual has a maximum heart rate of 170 beats per minute and a resting heart rate of 70 beats per minute, resulting in a heart rate of 100 beats per minute. Take 65 percent of the heart rate reserve, and in this example that number is 65. Add it to your resting heart rate (70 beats per minute). The lowest intensity of exercise you should perform is 135 beats per minute. The highest intensity would be 85 percent of the heart rate reserve, plus the resting heart rate or 150 beats per minute. The training heart rate is determined by the following formula: [(220-age)-resting heart rate] x intensity desired + resting heart rate. The intensity of 65 to 85 percent of heart rate reserve must be sustained for 30 to 45 minutes. This cannot be easily done with many activities, such as weight training, tennis, racquetball, or handball. In these activities the heart rate can go up to as high as 94 or 100 percent of maximum, but remain at that level for a short period of time, and then the heart rate may go down to 30 or 50 percent. Rope jumping and swimming is also very good cardiovascular exercises, but they too can be difficult to sustain at high intensity for 30 to 45 minutes. The trick is to find an activity that you enjoy and then try to meet the high intensity criteria.

D. Frequency of Exercise

How many times per week must this activity be performed to improve cardiovascular endurance? Research has shown that the optimal frequency is three to four alternate days per week. You can vary the activity from work out to workout as long as the intensity and duration are adequate. Dr. Kenneth Cooper has devised an easy test for cardiovascular endurance. It entails covering as much distance as you can in 12 minutes. He has established norms based on age and sex in his book Aerobics.

Once you have selected your activity and determined your training heart rate, an exercise regime should be established. Example: Fifteen to 20 minutes of warm up activities. These are usually stretching exercises for the back of the legs, lower and upper back, hips, and trunk area. Add to this some muscular strength and endurance exercises for the stomach and upper body muscles (push-ups, pull downs, curl ups, leg raises). Then do the aerobic portion of the regime. If you are just starting your exercise program, do 10 to 15 minutes of aerobic exercises until you are more cardiovascularly conditioned. After this do a 10 to 20 minute cool-down of slow jogging or walking, and flexibility exercises. Your heart rate should be well below 100 beats per minute at the end of this period. After an exercise program such as this, you will find yourself with more energy and feeling better about yourself, plus you will be losing any excess weight with no great dietary restrictions.

E. Muscular Endurance

Muscular endurance is the ability of a muscle group to lift a weight as many times as possible. The greater number of times this can be accomplished, the greater your muscular endurance. The muscles that need the most endurance work are the arm group, the shoulder group, and the abdominal group. The leg and back muscles get a large amount of endurance work merely through standing, walking, and any antigravity activities; they also are used in cardiovascular exercises, such as jogging, cycling, etc. Increasing the endurance of the arm, shoulder, and abdominal muscles will enable you to better perform other activities (work around the home, or office). You will also derive more enjoyment from those occasional sporting endeavors, such as golf, tennis, racquetball, volleyball, etc. without extreme soreness and tired muscles the next day.

Muscle endurance development requires just a few exercises, push-ups, pull-ups, curl-ups or crunch-ups, along with leg raises, if your back is in good shape, two or three times per week. Push-ups and pull-ups are very beneficial in increasing the endurance of the arm and shoulder groups. Twenty to 30 push-ups per day is usually adequate, however, if you're occupational or recreational pursuits require a large amount of arm and upper bodywork, more repetitions may be necessary. It may be difficult to find a place to perform pull-ups. Commercial bars that are designed to fit in a doorway can be purchased but if pull-ups cannot be performed merely hanging with bent arms will do wonders to improve upper body endurance. Curl-ups or crunch-ups should be performed.

F. Muscular Strength

Muscular strength, the ability to lift the greatest weight possible at one time, is being developed, to a certain degree, at the same time as muscular endurance. (If added strength is not needed, no other exercises besides those used for muscular endurance are required.) The exercises performed to increase muscular strength are those that place an increased resistance on movement. The key is to start with very lightweights and progress slowly. You can use a large book or household objects, such as a soup can, a barbell, or even your own body weight. Perform 10 to 20 repetitions of each exercise three times with a rest period of two to three minutes between sets. During the third set you should be fatigued and find it impossible to do the required 10 to 20 repetitions. If 20 repetitions can be performed on the last set then increase the weight 5 to 10 pounds.

G. Exercise Methods

1. Free-hand Methods:
Free-hand exercise can be done anywhere, anytime, and without expensive equipment. The following six exercises are designed to tone up the arms, chest, shoulders, back, thighs, and calves and to tighten and muscularize the abdomen. Before going into the exercise, a brief explanation of

terminology is required. In each exercise you will begin with a given number of repetitions ("reps") and sets.

Example: If you perform 10 push-ups without stopping that is 1 set of 10 reps

A. Leg Raises

This exercise warms up the muscles of the trunk and lower back and tends to trim the lower abdominal area. While lying on your back on the floor, with hands under the hips, raise the legs upward (with knees slightly bent), until the toes are pointing to the ceiling. Inhale as you lower the legs back to the starting position.

Don't let your feet touch the floor. Repeat for 10-12 reps.

Remember: Exhale as the legs are raised; inhale as they are lowered.

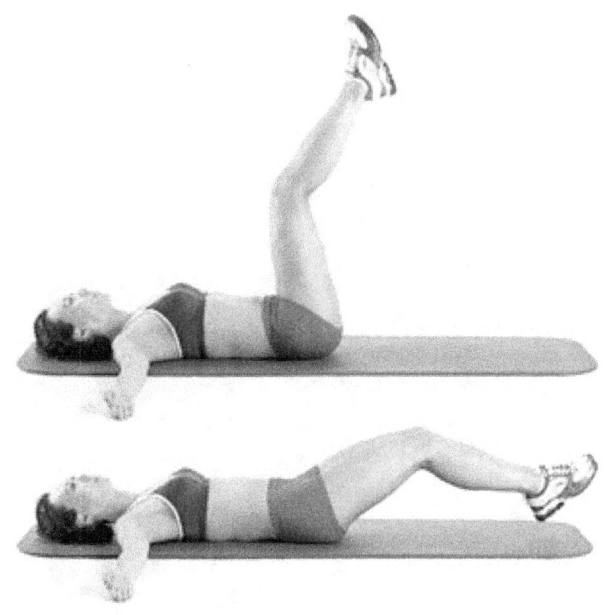

B. Crunch-Ups

This is another great abdominal exercise, working mostly the upper abdomen. Lie flat on the floor with the knees bent. It is more advantageous to keep the legs bent during this exercise because this puts all of the stress on the front abdominal muscles, rather than on the hip flexors. Exhale as you situp; inhale as you return to the starting position. Start with 6-12 reps until you're strong enough to do sets of 30. If you appear to have back pain discontinue.

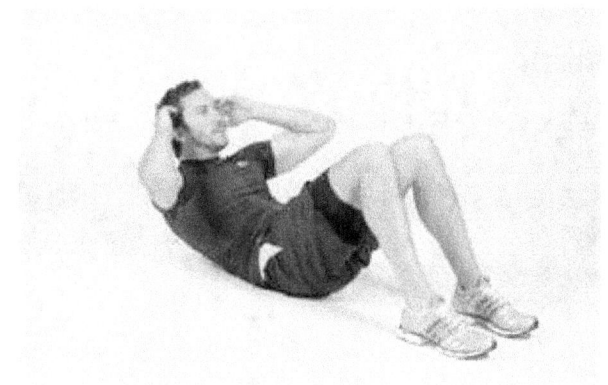

C. Push-ups

This is a great toner for the chest, shoulders, and the back of the arms, (triceps). Face down on the floor, keeping your hands about 18 inches apart (This exercise can be made more difficult by elevating the feet on a chair.) Start with arms extended. Inhale as you lower your chest until it touches the floor; exhale as you push up until your arms are straight. Start with 6-12 reps. If you can do more than 12, elevate your feet.

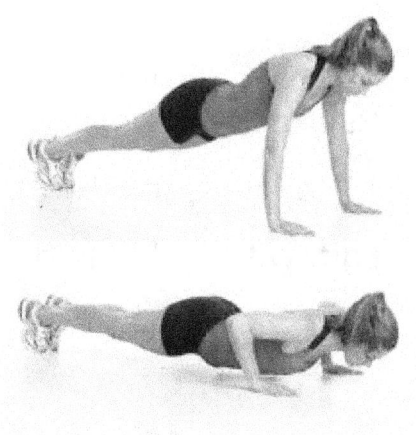

D. Chair Pull-ups

This exercise will help to develop the back and biceps. You'll need a sturdy pole and two chairs about 30-36 inches apart. Grasp the pole with an overhand grip; your hands should be about 24 to 30 inches apart. Keeping your body straight, feet stretched out in front of you, chest parallel to the pole, pull-up until your chest touches the pole, then slowly lower yourself, letting your back muscles stretch as you do so. This is a difficult exercise, so begin with 4-8 reps. Work up to 10-15. Exhale as you pullup; inhale as you lower your body.

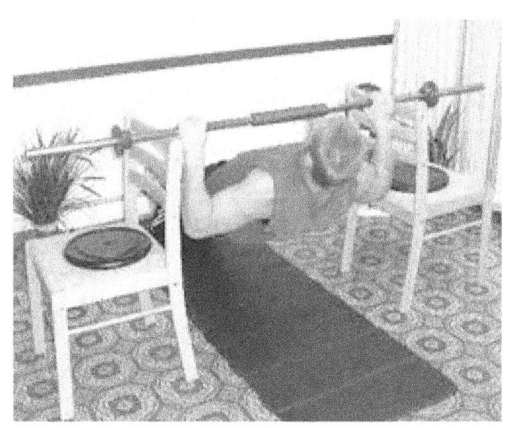

E. Dips

Dips are a great exercise to work the shoulders, the back of the arm (triceps), and the chest (pectorals). You should try to do 1 set of 10 to begin with. This is one of my favorite exercises.

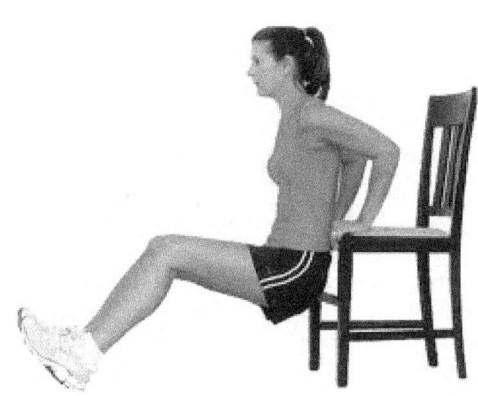

F. Deep Knee Bends (Squats)

This exercise builds and tones the thighs and strengthens the hips. With your feet about 18 inches apart and standing erect, squat down, keeping your back straight until your thighs are parallel to the floor. Inhale on the way down and exhale while returning to the starting position. Breathe deeply on this exercise and lift the chest up high on each inhalation. If you find it hard to maintain your balance, place a 2x4-inch block of wood under your heels. Begin with 6-12 reps. Work up to 20 reps.

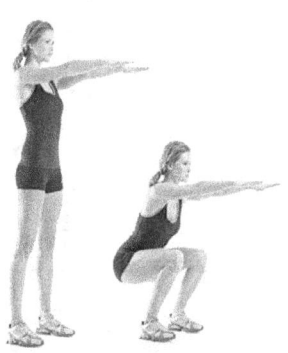

G. Indoor Jogging

In order to exercise the heart and lungs, endurance activities are required. Twenty to 40 minutes at the end of this exercise program should be devoted to aerobic exercise. If you cannot get outdoors to run, jog in place.

First, pick a location that will be comfortable for you like a soft, carpeted area. Purchase a jogging board, or treadmill and try to jog for 10 minutes. Then progress by 2-3 minute intervals until you're jogging for 30 minutes. Try to get your heart rate up to between 130 - 150 beats per minute. Regulate the stepping frequency and the height of your knee lift to achieve your desired heart rate.

Heart Rate Formula
[(220-age) – resting heart rate] x intensity desired + resting heart rate

---

Workout Program

If you are underweight and want to normalize your weight

and

build up your body, use the following program.

EXERCISE	SETS	REPS
Leg raises	1	Maximum
Sit-ups	1	Maximum
Dips	1	10
Push-ups	5	10-20
Chair pull-ups	5	10 – 15
Deep knee bends	4	15 – 25
Indoor jogging		20 – 40 min

Begin with one set of each exercise for four days the first week. (Monday, Tuesday, Thursday, Friday.) The second week, perform two sets of the push-ups, chair pull-ups, and deep knee bends. Rest about 1 ½ to 2 minutes between sets and exercises. The third week, you should be able to do the complete program.

If you want to trim down and lose body fat, alter the program as follows:

EXERCISE	SETS	REPS
Leg raises	5	20 – 40
Sit-ups	5	20 – 40
Dips	1	10-20
Push-ups	3	15 - 25
Chair pull-ups	3	10 – 15
Jogging		20 – 40 min

Workout four days per week as in the previous program, slowly building up to the complete workout.

If you are basically in good condition, and just want to maintain excellent body tone, use the following program:

EXERCISE	SETS	REPS
Leg raises	3	25 – 50
Sit-ups	3	25 – 50
Dips	1	20
Push-ups	3	20 - 40
Chair pull-ups	3	15 – 20
Jogging		20 – 40 min

Try to work out 4 days per week

2. Progressive Resistance Weight Training

This method of training requires equipment normally found in gyms—barbells, dumbbells, etc. Weight training is a wonderful way to stay in good shape, increase your strength, and reshape your body. The following program is basic for the average person who wants to stay in good condition.

EXERCISE	SETS	REPS
Deep knee bends/squats	3	8 – 10
Leg curls	3	8 – 10
Calf raises	3	12 – 15
Bench press	3	8 – 10
Incline dumbbell press	3	8 – 10
Flat flys	3	8 – 10
Behind the neck press	3	8 – 10
Side lateral raises	3	8 – 10
Pull-ups behind the neck	3	6 – 8
Stiff-leg dead lifts	3	6 – 8
French press	3	6 – 8
Press downs	3	8 – 10
Barbell curls	3	8 – 10
Crunch-Up	2	25
Leg raises	2	20

Exercise three days per week (Monday, Wednesday, Friday). Rest only 1 1/2 to 2 minutes between sets and exercises. When the reps become too easy, increase the resistance or weight. Begin the program slowly to avoid extreme muscle soreness. Some form of endurance training can be added to this program (jogging, bicycling, swimming, etc.).

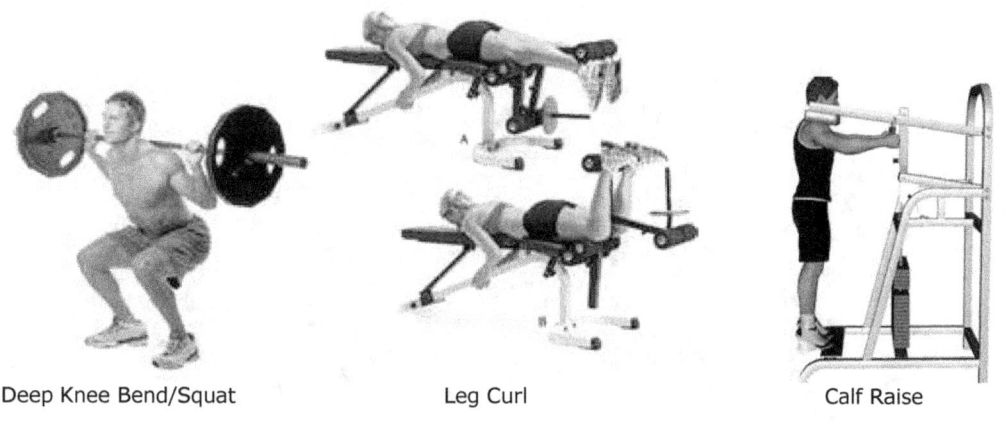

Deep Knee Bend/Squat   Leg Curl   Calf Raise

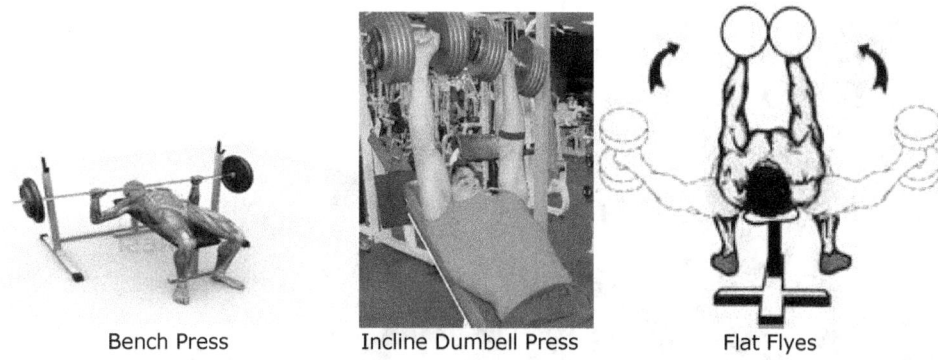

Bench Press   Incline Dumbell Press   Flat Flyes

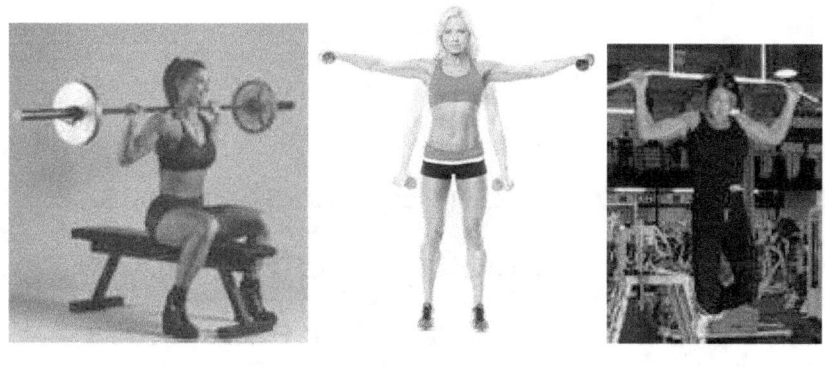

Behind Neck Press   Side Lateral Raises   Pull-Ups Behind Neck

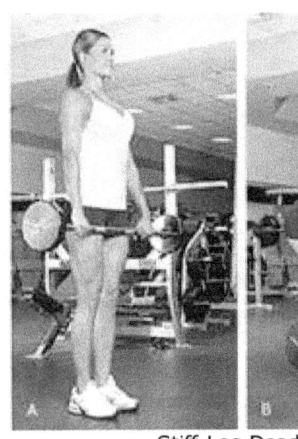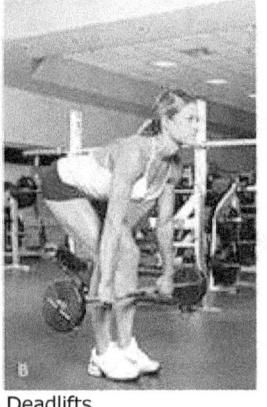

Stiff-Leg Deadlifts

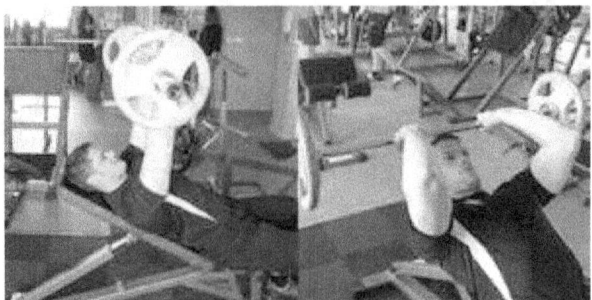

French Press

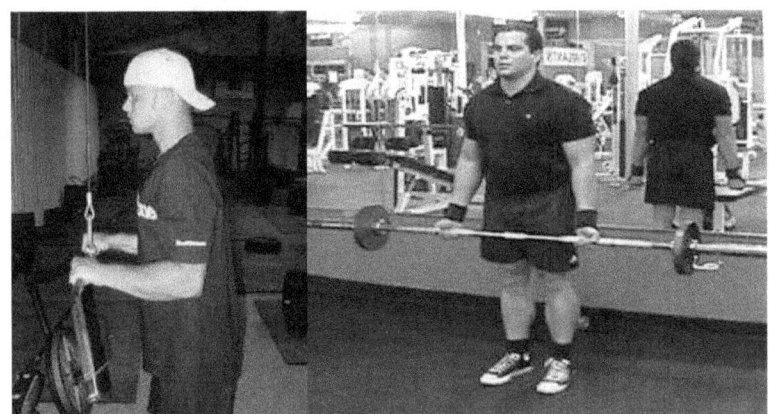

Press Downs   Barbell Curl

3.   Flexibility

Flexibility is the ability to move adjoining bone structures closer together or increase the range of movement around any joint structure. Bone and soft tissue structures limit much of flexibility; however, most individuals can improve their flexibility 100 percent if they work on it properly. The importance of increasing flexibility is two-fold. First, with increasing flexibility, the chances of injuries due to physical activity are reduced. Second, flexibility helps a person perform normal functions more efficiently. It can also help to reduce normal aches and pains. This is why it is recommended to stretch out before and after any activity. Yoga-type or Hatha yoga stretching exercises are very good. But no matter what style of stretching you perform a few tips should be followed:

Never bob or bounce when stretching. None of the movements should be sudden. Slow, easy, continuous stretching is much better than ballistic type movements.

Don't go beyond the point of pain or discomfort. Your body is trying to tell you something by evoking the pain receptors. Listen to it. When you feel pain or discomfort, ease up a little and hold the position as you relax. Extend the stretch again, very slowly, until the discomfort returns, then ease up a little and hold.

All stretches should be held for 10 to 30 seconds. This gives the muscles time to relax and get accustomed to the new position. When you finally relax, you will find you can extend the stretch without an unpleasant feeling. You should feel a slight strain or pull in the muscles and joints being stretched, but no pain. Flexibility exercises should be performed 10 to 20 minutes before and after the main exercise session. This is a hard habit to get into but it will be one of great benefit if it is followed routinely. If time does not permit adding the flexibility exercises directly onto the workout program, try doing the exercises at some other time that day, such as when you're watching TV or reading the newspaper.

An easy test to determine if your flexibility is up to par is to sit on the floor with your legs extended out in front of you and the bottoms of your feet are flat up against a wall. Lean forward, slowly, with your arms extended and try to touch your toes. If you can put your palms on the wall by your feet, your flexibility is excellent and you should continue to maintain it. If you can touch the wall with your fists you are considered average. However, you may be more likely to lose some of this flexibility if you don't work on it regularly. If you are just able to touch the wall with your fingertips or if you can't touch the wall at all, you need extra flexibility work. (If you can reach only to the middle of your shin, don't delay!) Start easy and remember: "Strain, no pain."

Exercises for Special Groups

1. Elderly

Age should not stop anyone from starting an exercise program but be sure to have a complete physical exam before beginning. Any orthopedic problems should be explored to determine if certain types of exercises are not recommended.

A swimming program can be most enjoyable and relaxing as well as a good conditioner for the body. If deep water is frightening to you, try walking in knee-deep water perhaps, gradually going into a little bit deeper water for added resistance. You can achieve the desired heart rate by varying the walking speed. (Water exercise takes the weight off the lower extremities and relieves stress in the lower back. Arms can be used to propel the body through the water as upper body exercise.) Light calisthenics and flexibility exercises can also be very beneficial and can help the individual to move their joints through a fuller range of motion. Tai Chi is an excellent exercise for the elderly, Also, many elderly people must watch their diets a little more closely because as people age their BMR declines and so does their caloric intake. If the wrong foods are ingested, a deficiency in some of the vitamins and nutrients can occur. This situation is compounded by the added demands of exercise, so be sure to supplement your diet with nutritious foods. Remember, though it would be an overstatement to say that people who exercise regularly will live longer, it's not an overstatement to say that they will feel better, derive more enjoyment out of life, and will grow old more gracefully than the people who don't exercise.

2. Pregnancies and Post Pregnancy

It has been well documented that women have exercised vigorously, jogged three miles and more per day, up to a week before delivery and have resumed running three days after being released from the hospital. I personally do not recommend that as a normal procedure for pregnancy. However, many doctors are realizing the benefits of regular exercise during pregnancy. In fact, many women state that their pregnancies were much easier when they exercised than when they were inactive. The critical thing to remember is not to start a vigorous exercise program **after** you find out that you are pregnant. If you have been exercising, and then you can continue, just be sure to listen to your body and discuss your exercise program with your doctor. It may be necessary to cut down on the amount or intensity of your exercising in the third trimester. When to stop exercising before delivery is up to you and your physician. The same rule dictates when to resume your exercise program after delivery.

3. Cardiac Rehabilitation

There is still quite a bit of controversy about exercise and the heart disease patient. Many hospitals have a Phase I program. This is a step-by-step rehabilitation program that begins about three days after the initial heart attack. It starts with very light range-of-motion exercises and gradually builds up to a walking program, which may include stair climbing at a slow, controlled rate. The Phase II program is started when the patient is discharged from the hospital. This is usually a bicycle program or a walking program. This phase may last 2 to 3 months. After this period, they can go into Phase III, the conditioning/maintenance period. I have observed cardiac patients who thought that they would never be able to resume enjoying the activities that they participated in before the heart attack lead a full and productive life after incorporating exercise into their therapy program. To find out if your community has such a program, contact your local cardiologist or hospital.

4.   Diabetic

Exercise has long been advocated for certain types of diabetic patients. It is, however not recommended for the poorly controlled or the uncontrolled diabetic. Recent research has shown that during exercise, diabetic's insulin receptors become more sensitive to insulin and therefore lead to a marked use in glucose utilization. It is very important for the diabetic to seek medical advice before increasing his/her activity level. If you are diabetic, you will probably have to regulate the amount of, exercise, caloric and intake medication very precisely. It will also be necessary to determine your regular glucose level until you achieve a good, balanced program. In general, each individual will have his/her own limitations and precautions while exercising. Keeping a candy bar, orange juice, or sugar cube handy may be a good idea for some diabetics.

5.   Hypertension /High Blood Pressure

It is estimated that over 23 million individuals in the United States are considered to be hypertensive. High blood pressure has been called the "silent killer" because there are no overt symptoms that can warn the individual that an abnormality is present. Often the hypertension leads to heart disease and kidney problems before they are diagnosed. When diagnosed in its early stages, hypertension is difficult to treat, not because there aren't medications but rather that the patient will not stick to advised treatment. (It is difficult to take medication daily when there are no symptoms or feelings of discomfort. In fact, the blood pressure medication may make the person feel worse.) It has been suggested that exercise can lower blood pressure; however, hypertension should be controlled before beginning an exercise program.

It is estimated that many millions of individuals in the United States are considered to be hypertensive. High blood pressure has been called the "silent killer" because there are no overt symptoms that can warn the individual that an abnormality is present. Often the hypertension leads to heart disease and kidney problems before they are diagnosed. When diagnosed in its early stages, hypertension is difficult to treat, not because there aren't medications but rather that the patient will not stick to advised treatment. (It is difficult to take medication daily when there are no symptoms or feelings of discomfort. In fact, the blood pressure medication may make the person feel worse.) It has been suggested that exercise can lower blood pressure; however, hypertension should be controlled before beginning an exercise program.

6.   Obesity

Being obese is a real problem when trying to exercise. It has become almost epidemic in our young. The added weight makes all movement less efficient and more difficult. Therefore, the obese person should begin with a very light exercise program accompanied by a moderate diet. Remember if you diet without exercising, lean body weight or muscle tissue will be lost as well as fat. Also, the BMR will fall and it will take fewer calories to supply energy for the body at rest. Exercise and dieting will cause an increase in BMR and a good portion of the weight lost will be fat. The exercise I recommend is walking. The caloric expenditure for walking or jogging a certain distance is the same.

SPEED	KCAL/MIN/KG	KCAL/MIN	KCAL 170LB PERSON
Walking 19 min/mile	0.080	1.52	117.04
Jogging 11.5 min/mile	0.135	1.55	119.35
Jogging 6 min/mile	0.252	1.51	116.27

You can see that the caloric costs for walking and jogging are about the same. However, the cardiovascular conditioning effect will probably be a lot less at the very low walking speeds.

Caloric Expenditure as a Result of Exercise

Body composition is of importance in total fitness. Extra weight in the form of fat decreases efficiency and makes the body, work harder to perform a given amount of work. This extra work also makes the heart work harder. The value of proper nutrition in controlling body weight has been well stated throughout this book and if the guidelines set forth is followed; they could go a long way to help correct the problem of obesity. However, the simple fact remains that you consume more calories then you burn up, you will gain weight. It doesn't matter if the extra calories are in the form of protein, carbohydrates, or fat. If you consume an extra 3,500 kcal of lettuce, a pound of fat will be gained just the same as if you consumed 3,500 extra kcal of chocolate cake. It is much easier to cut out 500 kcal per day dieting and exercise off another 500 kcal per day than it is to cut out

1,000 kcal per day dieting. What activities do I recommend for weight loss or control? Any physical activity will increase the metabolism rate and thereby the body will burn more calories when at rest. Some exercises are better than others. Weight lifting, sit-ups, push-ups and other muscular strength and endurance exercises will cause an increase in the metabolic rate; however, these activities only last 30 seconds to one minute. Long periods of continuous exercise will be most beneficial for weight loss. So if you decrease your caloric intake by 400 kcal per day and walk 3 miles per day, which expends 350 kcal, you will have expended 750 kcal more than you consumed.   This would enable you to lose 1 and one half pounds per week—more than an adequate weight loss rate. In six months, you could see a 36-pound loss. With only a five-day per week walking program you could lose about a pound per week and 52 pounds in a year. There are quicker ways to lose weight, but 95 percent of the time there is a corresponding quick weight return.

How can you tell if you are obese? There are a few scientific methods, such as underwater weight, and electronic or skin fold measurements but unless you have access to a human performance laboratory, YMCA, YWCA, or a university, these methods are probably not available to you. But most overweight people know that they are carrying around more weight than is necessary. The mirror is the best indicator.

When you're home alone, stand in front of a full-length mirror, take a paper bag and cut out two small holes for your eyes and place the bag over your head. Now take off all your clothes. It's much easier to be "objective" when there's no face connected to the body. The pinch test is also useful. If you can pinch an inch or more of fat around your waist, it's time to watch what you eat and begin to exercise.

Fitness and Longevity

Probably the greatest reward you can achieve by following the increase in Physical Fitness is an increase in longevity. Not only can you improve your fitness and well being, but also you can gain the increased time to enjoy this new lifestyle. A landmark study by the Institute for Aerobics Research and the Cooper Clinic Study on Fitness and Longevity (1989) that tracked the fitness and health of more than 13,000 men and women over an eight-year period, indicates that even moderate exercise can lower death rates, including those from cancer. The Dallas based institute and clinic began the study by measuring the fitness levels of each subject with a maximal treadmill exercise test. The subjects were then divided into five fitness categories ranging from healthy but sedentary to the serious athlete, such as people who ran 30 to 40 miles per week. Eight years after the original testing, 240 men and 43 women had died. After accounting for other risk factors, such as smoking, high cholesterol, high blood pressure, diabetes, and family history, researchers showed that a high percentage of the deaths came from the least fit group. Least-fit males died 3.5 times more than the fit male and the least-fit female died 4.5 times more than her counterpart. (Even cancer deaths were higher for the least-fit group.) The most unexpected result was the difference in death rates between the least-fit group and the next to least-fit. The group of males with only moderate fitness levels had almost a third fewer deaths than their sedentary counterparts. In fact, the study reported that poor fitness is an important risk factor for all causes of mortality in both males and females. According to the data they collected, an unfit male could reduce his death risk by 37 percent if he became fit. The good news they reported is that you don't need to be a glutton for punishment to minimize the fitness level risk factor. A regular visit to a health club, golf club, tennis court, etc., can dramatically reduce your risk.

About the Author

Stanley Morey, Ph.D. is an accomplished author, writing many books in the bodybuilding and nutrition areas. He received his B.S. from the University of Tampa, attended J. Hillis Miller Medical School in Gainesville, and the University of South Florida, in Tampa. He received his Ph. D. from the University of the Pacific in 1972 in Physiology.

He was also a competitive bodybuilder for many years, winning many local and regional competitions as well as owning a successful health club for over 20 years.

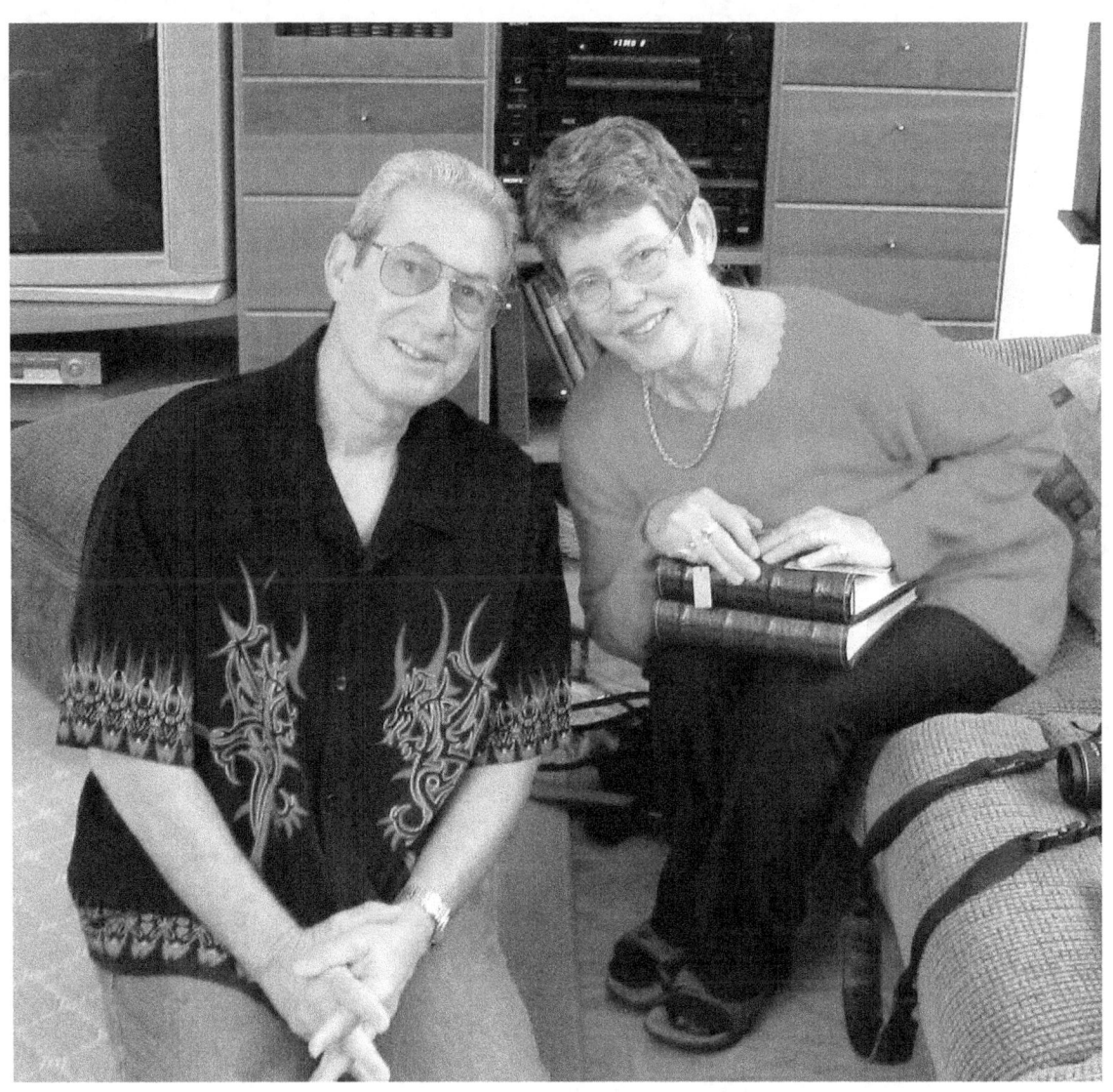

Author Stanley W. Morey, Ph.D. and wife Gery Morey